# CCM Certification Made Easy

Mickey Smith

## Blood Count

A common test that can assist in the diagnosis of numerous infections, diseases, and illnesses is the full blood count, or FBC. Using a needle inserted into a vein in your hand or the crook of your elbow, the doctor, nurse, or technician collects a sample of your blood.

The blood test is gathered inside an exceptional vial that contains a substance to keep the blood from coagulating. A machine and the sample are taken to a laboratory for analysis. Abnormalities in your blood, such as an unusually high or low number of blood cells, are looked for by the FBC test. If a problem is found, your doctor will usually order more tests to figure out what's wrong.

# Blood Count Method

Much of the time, no extraordinary planning is required before the test. The system regularly incorporates the accompanying:

You will be asked to sit or lie down at the surgery.

In order to increase the volume of blood in your veins, a tourniquet is placed around your arm and tightened. The specialist, attendant or professional might request that you hold and unclench your clench hand to assist enlarge your veins with blood.

An alcohol preparation is used to clean the injection site and lower the risk of infection.

The specialist, medical caretaker or expert embeds a needle into your vein and draws the blood, which is gathered inside a needle or vial. You might encounter some distress during the methodology, yet this is typically negligible.

The person taking the blood sample will ask you to apply gauze or cotton wool to the injection site to prevent bleeding after it has been taken. A dressing with adhesive will be applied to the injection site. For a few days, you may experience some minor bruising at the injection site.

Blood made sense of roughly seven to eight percent of your body weight is blood. This implies an individual who weighs 70 kg has roughly 5 to 5.5 liters of blood.

There are four main parts to blood. Plasma, which is a liquid made up of water, fat, protein, sugar, and salts, accounts for 60% of the total. The remaining 40% are blood cells, which include:

erythrocytes, also known as red blood cells, The oxygen-carrying protein known as haemoglobin is found in every red blood cell. Iron is found in haemoglobin, which is necessary for the white blood cells, also known as leukocytes, to transport oxygen throughout the body. These are infection-fighting immune system cells. Lymphocytes, eosinophils, monocytes, neutrophils, and basophils are the various types of white blood cells.

Platelets - help to cluster the blood to quit dying.

Blood serves a variety of purposes, including: transporting oxygen and nutrients to the tissues, forming blood clots to stop bleeding, transporting white blood cells and antibodies to fight infection, and transporting waste products to the liver and kidneys, which help filter and clean the blood.

## Assessment of the Full Blood Count

The full blood count test:

measures the average size of the red cells (mean cell volume) if necessary, reviews the blood cells under a microscope (blood smear/film), determines the ratio of red cells to plasma ('haematocrit' or 'packed cell volume'), counts the total number of white cells, platelets, and red blood cells in the sample, and determines the count of each of the white cell subsets.

## Irregularities in a Full Blood Count

The consequences of a full blood count are contrasted with graphs that rundown the typical scope of numbers and proportions for each kind of platelet. A possible abnormality is a result that is either above or below the normal range.

Numerous sicknesses, illnesses or contaminations other than the ones recorded beneath can cause a strange full blood count result. The sample of blood may have abnormalities such as:

**Red platelets and hemoglobin** - low levels (sickliness) may recommend insufficient iron in the eating regimen, blood misfortune or certain persistent illnesses (like kidney illness). Significant levels (polycythaemia) may propose polycythaemia vera, kidney sickness, constant lung illness or physiological changes because of living in areas of high height

**Red platelet to plasma proportion** - a lower-than-typical proportion of red platelets to plasma proposes the individual might have sickliness. The contrary finding proposes that the individual might be dried out or has such a large number of red cells (polycythaemia)

**White platelets** - low levels (leucopenia) may propose the individual has a viral contamination, bone marrow sickness or has been presented to chemo-or radiotherapy. Low levels (thrombocytopenia) may be the result of taking certain medications, a viral infection, bone marrow disorders, or an autoimmune disorder. High levels (leucocytosis) may indicate a bacterial infection, an inflammatory disease, or a bone marrow disease. High levels (thrombocythaemia) may indicate the presence of an inflammatory condition or bone marrow disease.

Blood smear When your blood sample is examined under a microscope, it is called a "blood smear."

## A smear of blood can reveal:

A scope of infections including red platelet problems (like sickle cell frailty)

The presence of blood-borne parasites like jungle fever

A white platelet problem like lymphoma or leukemia.

## Full Blood Count and Exactness

The full blood count test isn't secure and mistakes now and again happen. Your doctor will want to do the test again if this happens. Errors could be:

Disappointment of the gear - for instance, the blood coagulations in the vial

Wrong naming of the example

Wrong treatment of the example - for instance the example is left in the sun and weakens

Tainting of the example

Liquor in the blood.

A blood test known as a complete blood count (CBC) is one. It gives your supplier data about your blood and generally speaking wellbeing. A wide range of diseases, conditions, disorders, and infections can be diagnosed, monitored, and screened for with the assistance of CBCs. Your supplier takes an example of blood and your lab results are generally prepared inside a couple of days.

## What exactly is a CBC (complete blood count)?

A blood test is a complete blood count (CBC). It assists medical professionals in identifying a variety of conditions and disorders. Additionally, it looks for signs of medication side effects in your blood. Suppliers utilize this test to evaluate for sicknesses and change therapies.

Your blood cells are counted and measured in a CBC. A blood sample is taken from you by your doctor and sent to a lab. In order to evaluate your blood cells, the lab conducts a series of tests. These tests assist your supplier with checking your wellbeing.

## When is a CBC performed?

You might require a CBC on the off chance that you have side effects, for example,

Bleeding or bruising

Weariness, dazedness or shortcoming.

Vertigo, nausea, and fever.

Aggravation (expanding and bothering) anyplace in the body.

Pain in the joints

issues with blood pressure or heart rate.

Why are CBCs ordered by healthcare providers?

An essential component of a yearly physical examination are CBCs. CBCs are also ordered by providers to keep track of the side effects of some prescription drugs.

## Your Supplier Might Arrange A CBC To:

Recognize anomalies in your blood that might be indications of illness.

Numerous disorders, conditions, and infections can be diagnosed or monitored.

Assess your general wellbeing.

Eliminate diseases, disorders, and conditions.

Screen different blood illnesses.

## What Criteria Does A CBC Use?

Numerous tests to measure and study platelets, white blood cells, and red blood cells are performed during a CBC. Oxygen is carried throughout the body by red blood cells. Your immune system includes white blood cells. They assist your body with battling contamination. Platelets aid in blood clotting.

Numerous aspects of your blood are counted, evaluated, and studied by a CBC:

The total number of white blood cells is counted using a CBC without a differential.

Differential in CBC. White blood cells come in five different varieties. The differential examines your total number of each type of white blood cell.

Tests for hemoglobin measure hemoglobin, the oxygen-carrying protein in red blood cells.

The amount of red blood cells in your blood is referred to as your hematocrit.

Your provider is informed by a CBC:

how many brand-new blood cells are being produced by your body.

The total number of platelets, white blood cells (WBC), and red blood cells (RBC, also known as erythrocytes).

Dimensions and form of blood cells

A CBC detects what?

A CBC blood test can assist your supplier with diagnosing many circumstances, problems, sicknesses and contaminations, including:

Weakness (when there aren't sufficient red platelets to bring oxygen through the body).

Bone marrow issues, for example, myelodysplastic conditions.

Issues like agranulocytosis and thalassemias and sickle cell pallor.

White blood cell counts that are abnormally low or high due to infections or other issues

a variety of cancers, including lymphoma and leukemia.

Results of chemotherapy and a few professionally prescribed prescriptions.

Mineral and vitamin deficiencies

Details of the test: What can I anticipate from a complete blood count (CBC)?

There is nothing you need to do to prepare for a CBC. A needle is inserted and your arm is cleaned by your provider. The needle shouldn't hurt, though it might sting or pinch a little. The needle is typically inserted into the baby's heel by caregivers.

A portion of your blood is taken out of you with a needle and collected in a tube. Occasionally, your physician will require multiple blood tubes

Your doctor will remove the needle and apply a bandage to your arm after drawing blood. Your supplier sends the blood to a lab. Your blood supply is quickly restored.

What can I anticipate following the exam?

On your arm, tape will hold a bandage and some gauze in place. For a few hours, your arm may be a little sore. You might get a small bruise where your doctor put the needle in.

## What advantages does this test provide?

Your doctor can get a picture of your overall health from a CBC. A CBC can assist in the detection of hundreds of conditions, disorders, and infections by utilizing a small amount of blood. It lets your doctor keep an eye on your health, check for diseases, and plan and change your treatment.

## What are this test's potential dangers?

A CBC is a common, safe test. Your provider will only remove a small amount of blood, so there are no risks. After a CBC, some people occasionally experience lightheadedness or fainting.

## Results and Consultation

Results are typically prepared inside a couple of days. Some of the time it just requires 24 hours to come by results. Your provider will get in touch with you to talk about the next steps and explain the results. On the off chance that your platelet counts are beyond the typical reach, your supplier might arrange follow-up tests.

**For a complete blood count, what are the usual ranges?**

Normal hemoglobin range:

Males over 15: 13.0- 17.0 g/dL Females over the age of 15: The normal range for hematocrit is 11.5-15.5 g/dL:

Male: 40-55% are women: 36 - 48%

Platelet Count ordinary reach:

Adult: 150,000 - 400,000/mL

White platelet (WBC) typical reach:

Adult: 5,000-10,000/mL When do I need to see a doctor?

The outcomes of your CBC will be discussed with you by your provider. Call your service provider if you have any questions about the results.

Complete blood counts are used by healthcare providers to treat illness and maintain health. With one example of blood, CBCs can help screen for many problems, conditions and diseases. A complete blood count (CBC) can identify conditions early, sometimes before symptoms appear, allowing for prompt treatment. CBCs are a fundamental device in keeping up with great generally speaking wellbeing.

A total blood count (CBC) is a blood test. It is utilized to examine one's overall health and identify a wide variety of conditions, such as leukemia, infection, and anemia.

A total blood count test estimates the accompanying:

Hemoglobin, the oxygen-carrying protein in red blood cells, Hematocrit, the amount of red blood cells in the blood, Platelets, which aid in blood clotting, and white blood cells, which fight infection. A complete blood count can show unusual increases or decreases in cell counts. Those alterations may indicate a medical condition that necessitates additional testing.

## Why it's finished

A total blood count is a typical blood test accomplished for some reasons:

To examine one's overall health. A complete blood count can be part of a medical exam to check for conditions like anemia or leukemia as well as general health.

To make a medical diagnosis. A total blood count can assist with finding the reason for side effects like shortcoming, weakness and fever. Additionally, it may assist in determining the cause of pain, swelling, bruising, or bleeding.

To mind an ailment. A total blood count can assist with watching out for conditions that influence platelet counts.

to see how treatment is going. A complete blood count can be used to monitor radiation and medications that affect blood cell counts.

How to prepare: If the test is only for a complete blood count, you can eat and drink normally before the test. You might need to fast for a certain amount of time prior to the test if your blood sample will also be used for other tests. Find out what you need to do from your doctor.

What to expect During a complete blood count, a member of the healthcare team inserts a needle into a vein in your arm, typically at the bend of your elbow, to collect a sample of your blood. A laboratory receives the blood sample. You can immediately resume your usual activities following the test.

A complete blood count, also known as a CBC, is not a test that can definitively diagnose a condition. Results outside the normal reach might require follow-up. In addition to a CBC, a doctor might also need to look at the results of other tests.

For instance, results somewhat outside the regular reach on a CBC probably won't be of worry for somebody who's solid and has no side effects of disease. There may not be a need for follow-up. However, if a CBC results outside the expected range for a person undergoing treatment for cancer, it may indicate that the treatment needs to be altered.

At times, for results that are way above or beneath the normal ranges, a medical care supplier could request that you see a specialist who treats blood problems, called a hematologist.

## What the Outcomes Might Demonstrate

Brings about the accompanying regions above or underneath the normal reaches on a total blood count could highlight an issue.

Hematocrit, hemoglobin, and the number of red blood cells. Because they each measure a characteristic of red blood cells, the results of these three are related.

Anemia is indicated by lower-than-usual results in these three areas. There are numerous causes of anemia. They might be caused by a lack of certain vitamins or iron, bleeding, or another health issue. Anemia can cause a person to feel tired and weak. These side effects might be because of the iron deficiency itself or the reason for paleness.

Erythrocytosis is characterized by a higher-than-normal number of red blood cells. A medical condition like blood cancer or heart disease may be indicated by a high red blood cell count, high hemoglobin, or high hematocrit levels.

Count of white blood cells. Leukopenia is a low white blood cell count. The cause could be a medical condition like an autoimmune disorder that kills white blood cells, problems with the bone marrow, or cancer. White blood cell counts can also fall when taking certain medications.

A white platelet count that is higher than expected most usually is because of a disease or irritation. Or on the other hand it could highlight an insusceptible framework issue or a bone marrow sickness. A reaction to medication or vigorous exercise can also result in a high white blood cell count.

**Count of platelets.** Thrombocytopenia is characterized by a lower-than-normal platelet count. It is referred to as thrombocytosis if it is higher than usual. Either can be a side effect of medication or a sign of a medical condition. If your platelet count falls outside the normal range, you probably need more tests to figure out what's wrong.

Medical tests that look for changes in chromosomes, genes, or proteins are known as genetic testing. To determine a person's genetic health, genetic tests examine a person's DNA in a variety of ways. They are all made to find a specific gene that could be the cause of a genetic disorder.

Our cells contain 46 chromosomes for each of us. DNA, or deoxyribonucleic acid, is the building block of chromosomes. Qualities are short segments of DNA and every chromosome contains hundreds to thousands of qualities. Our bodies need information from our genes to make proteins, which are chemicals. Proteins are essential to the processes that keep us alive and form the body's structure. The distinctions in our qualities makes us all people. A mutation occurs when a gene undergoes a change that either causes or increases the risk of a disease or disorder.

Note: the data underneath is a general aide in particular. There may be differences between hospitals in terms of how things are set up and how tests are done. Always adhere to your doctor's or local hospital's instructions.

## What Are Chromosomes, DNA, And Genes?

Your body is comprised of millions of little cells. Various kinds of cells structure the various designs of the body, including skin, muscles, nerves and furthermore organs like the liver and kidneys.

The DNA molecule is packaged into structures that look like threads and are called chromosomes in the center (nucleus) of most cells in your body. 23 pairs of 46 chromosomes make up your genome. One pair of sex chromosomes (XX for females or XY for males) is included in these. Autosomes are the other chromosomes that do not determine whether we are male or female. There are 22 autosome pairs, ranging in number from 1 to 22. Your father and mother each give you one chromosome from each pair.

The fundamental component of your genetic material is a gene. It is comprised of a succession (or piece) of DNA and sits at a specific put on a chromosome. Therefore, a gene is a small chromosome segment. In your body, each gene controls a specific feature or performs a specific function. For instance, determining your eye or hair color, making all of your body's proteins, and so on. A pair is made up of each gene. Your father and mother each pass on one gene from each pair to you. There are hundreds of genes on each chromosome. There are between 20,000 and 25,000 genes in total in humans. Your genome is the sum of all of your genes.

Deoxyribonucleic acid is referred to as DNA. Your genetic material is made of DNA. Qualities, which are comprised of DNA, go about as guidelines to make proteins. In people, qualities fluctuate in size from only a tiny measure of DNA to exceptionally a lot of DNA.

Proteins are big, complicated molecules that your body uses for a lot of important things. They do a large portion of the work in cells and are expected for the construction, capability and guideline of your body's tissues and organs.

As our cells are duplicating constantly, our hereditary data needs to remain something similar. In most cases, excellent mechanisms ensure that each cell receives the same copy of our genes' material known as DNA. However, your genetic material may experience other issues or the copying mechanism may make mistakes at times. Gene abnormalities and problems can result in genetic diseases.

## What Is Hereditary Trying?

A medical test called genetic testing looks for changes in proteins, genes, or chromosomes. DNA taken from a person's blood, tissues, or other bodily fluids is examined for abnormalities in gene tests. The tests can search for huge errors, for example, a quality that has a segment missing or added.

Different tests search for little changes inside the DNA. Different slip-ups that can be found incorporate qualities that are excessively dynamic, qualities that are switched off, or those that are lost completely.

Hereditary tests look at an individual's DNA in various ways. They are undeniably intended to distinguish contrasts between the quality being tried and what might be viewed as an ordinary variant of a similar quality.

There are various kinds of genetic testing, including:

Atomic hereditary tests (or quality tests)

These gander at single qualities or short lengths of DNA taken from an individual's blood or other body liquids (for instance, spit) to recognize enormous changes, for example,

A gene in which a portion is missing or added; or minor modifications, such as a DNA strand component that is absent, added, or altered.

Genetic testing, on the other hand, has some drawbacks because it is only useful if it is known that a particular genetic mutation causes a particular condition. The DNA undergoes a permanent change as a result of a mutation or error in the copying process, which can lead to a variety of diseases. Huntington's disease, for instance, is known to be caused by a specific gene mutation. Therefore, a blood sample can be tested to determine whether or not this gene mutation is present. There may be any one of hundreds or even thousands of distinct gene mutations for a variety of conditions, including diabetes. As a result, genetic testing for those conditions is almost nonexistent.

Chromosomal genetic tests examine a person's chromosomes, their structure, number, and arrangement, among other things. A chromosome can have parts that are missing, extra, or even moved to a different part on another chromosome.

**There are a variety of approaches to chromosome testing.**

These are some:

Karyotyping is a test that produces a picture of a person's entire chromosome array. It is able to determine changes in the number of chromosomes (such as Down's syndrome, which has an extra chromosome 21).

Fluorescent in situ hybridization (FISH) analysis is a test that looks at specific parts of the chromosomes. This test can find very small parts of the chromosomes that are either missing or extra (like in Duchenne muscular dystrophy, for example).

## Biochemical Tests

Biochemical tests check out at the sums or exercises of key proteins. Because genes contain the DNA code for making proteins, protein activity or levels that are abnormal can indicate that genes are not functioning normally. The screening of newborn babies frequently makes use of these kinds of tests. A metabolic condition, such as phenylketonuria, that affects one of the many essential chemical reactions in the body can be detected through biochemical screening, for instance.

## Types of Genetic Tests

The results of genetic tests can help determine a person's likelihood of developing or passing on a genetic disorder, as well as confirm or rule out a suspected genetic condition. In excess of 2,000 hereditary tests are as of now being used, and more are being fostered constantly.

Hereditary testing is acted in various ways including:

The purpose of newborn screening is to identify genetic conditions that can be treated early in life. For instance, the heel prick test is used to check for cystic fibrosis in every newborn in the United Kingdom.

## Analytic Testing

Demonstrative testing is utilized to recognize or preclude a particular hereditary problem in the event that a child or individual has side effects to recommend a specific hereditary problem (for instance, Down's disorder).

## Testing For Carriers

Carriers are people who have one copy of a gene mutation—a genetic change—that, when present in two copies, results in a genetic disorder (such as sickle cell disease). Carriers can be identified through carrier testing. A test of this kind can be helpful in determining a couple's likelihood of having a child with a genetic disorder.

Testing before pregnancy (prenatal) is used to find changes in the genes of an unborn child.

If there is an increased risk that the baby will have a genetic or chromosomal disorder, this kind of testing is offered during pregnancy. However, it is unable to identify all potential inherited disorders and birth defects.

## Pre-Implantation Testing

Pre-implantation hereditary testing is accessible for couples who are in danger of having a kid with a particular hereditary or chromosome jumble, eg cystic fibrosis, sickle cell illness or Huntington's infection.

After egg cells are removed from the woman's ovaries, sperm cells outside the body fertilize the eggs. In-vitro fertilization, or IVF, is the term for this procedure. To produce embryos, sperm cells are used to fertilize the eggs. The prepared undeveloped organisms create for three days and afterward a couple of cells are eliminated from every undeveloped organism.

The genetic material (DNA and chromosomes) extracted from the cells is examined for the inherited disorder. After that, one or two of the unaffected embryos are brought into the mother's uterus. In the event that the pregnancy is effective, the child won't be impacted by the turmoil it was tried for.

Predictive testing Predictive testing is a method for identifying genetic mutations linked to conditions that manifest after birth, frequently in later life. These tests can be useful to individuals who have a relative with a hereditary problem however who have no elements of the actual issue at the difficult period (for instance, bosom disease related with the BRCA1 quality). A person's risk of developing disorders with a genetic basis, such as certain types of cancer, can be identified with predictive testing.

A person's risk of developing a genetic disorder like haemochromatosis before they show any signs or symptoms can also be determined through testing. Families with a high genetic disease risk must endure uncertainty regarding their own and their children's futures.

A sense of relief can come from a genetic test finding that a person does not have a known gene mutation that is the cause of a certain disease. However, if there is no known treatment, a positive result may have a devastating impact on a person's life.

Anyway for certain issues a positive outcome might assist you with considering choices to forestall the problem. Women with BRAC1, for instance, are more likely to develop breast cancer and may choose to undergo breast enlargement surgery (mastectomy) or take tamoxifen to lower their risk. For more details, refer to the separate brochure on breast cancer.

Therefore, a specialist must carefully discuss with you your risks of being affected by the disorder, how the disorder would affect you, and the advantages and disadvantages of having a genetic test for the disorder prior to predictive testing. See the segment on hereditary guiding underneath.

DNA sequences are used in forensic testing to identify a person for legal purposes. Dissimilar to the tests portrayed above, legal testing isn't utilized to recognize quality transformations related with illness. Additionally, this kind of testing can be used to determine a child's paternity. Criminological testing can likewise be utilized for distinguishing human remaining parts when ID is unimaginable by different means - for instance, after a catastrophic event like a fire or torrent.

## How Are Genetic Tests Carried Out?

A blood or tissue sample is typically taken as part of genetic testing. This typically involves drawing blood from a vein in adults and children. Samples of saliva or a swab taken from the inside of your mouth can be used for some genetic tests.

In pregnancy, an example might be taken from the child by amniocentesis or chorionic villus examining. A sample of the liquid (amniotic fluid) that surrounds a baby is taken during amniocentesis. The procedure involves inserting a needle through the abdomen and into the uterus. A portion of the placenta is taken as a sample during chorionic villus testing. This is either finished by embedding a needle into the mid-region like in amniocentesis or by placing a slender cylinder into the neck of the belly (cervix). There is only a very small chance that you will miscarry as a result of either test. If you are offered these tests, your doctor will explain the risks so you can decide whether or not to have them.

Lately the Agreement test has opened up. This can be utilized during pregnancy and is finished utilizing an example of the mother's blood, so there is no gamble of premature delivery as there is with amniocentesis or chorionic villus examining.

As part of a newborn's heel prick test at around 5 days old, routine screening for genetic disorders like phenylketonuria is done.

The sample is taken and sent to the laboratory for analysis.

## How Long Does It Take To Test For Genetics?

All of the tests' results might not come back for weeks or even months. This varies based on the kind of genetic test that you have had. Your PCP ought to exhort you how long the outcomes will be.

## What Dangers Do The Home Testing Kits Pose?

Individually, you can purchase a number of genetic tests, many of which are now available online. Most of these tests require you to slice the inside of your cheek to collect some cells for testing. Doctors do not recommend these. If you test positive for a genetic disorder for which there is no treatment, many tests can make you feel even more anxious. If you don't have any other risk factors, they might also test you for diseases that you might never actually get. A positive BRAC1 gene test, for instance, does not guarantee that you will develop breast cancer in the future.

Consider whether you are ready to make lifestyle adjustments in light of the test results before you take any of these tests. These tests may not be very helpful to you if you are unwilling to take steps like quitting smoking or getting more exercise.

Additionally, many of these tests are unreliable and may produce extremely misleading results. You should discuss this in greater detail with your doctor if you want to be tested for a genetic disorder.

## How Does Genetic Counseling Work?

Because the information obtained from genetic testing can have a significant impact on your life, you may be referred to a genetic counselor. Genetic counseling is available to anyone who is currently undergoing genetic testing or is considering doing so. Hereditary directing is certainly not a mental treatment. Its goal is to give you all the information you need to decide if a genetic test is right for you.

**Information about: may be included in genetic counseling.**

The repercussions of a positive genetic disorder test, such as its psychological impact and other effects.

Whether or not to inform family members of your intention to take the test.

The standard example of movement of the illness you are being tried for and its likely medicines.

The data is given such that will permit you to pursue your own choice. Only you can choose the path that is best for you. The directing is vital for ensure you have all the significant data you really want to settle on the choice.

**People are influenced by the following when considering their options:**

The possibility of disease transmission.

The seriousness of an issue.

The possibility of receiving a diagnosis prior to birth

Religious, social, and moral convictions

You can also get post-test counseling to help you deal with the results of the test.

In a nutshell, genetic testing entails looking at your DNA, the chemical database that contains instructions for how your body works. Changes or mutations in your genes that could lead to illness or disease can be discovered through genetic testing.

Albeit hereditary testing can give significant data to diagnosing, treating and forestalling disease, there are limits. For instance, even if you're in good health, a positive genetic test result doesn't always mean you'll get sick. However, a negative test result does not always mean you will not have a particular disorder.

An important part of getting genetic testing done is talking to your doctor, a medical geneticist, or a genetic counselor about what you'll do with the results.

Genome sequencing is the process of analyzing a sample of DNA taken from your blood when genetic testing does not result in a diagnosis but a genetic cause is still suspected. Some facilities offer genome sequencing.

The DNA that is found in every one of a person's genes makes up their individual genome. This sophisticated testing can assist in locating genetic variants that may have an impact on your health. Most of the time, these tests only look at the parts of DNA that make proteins, called the exome.

Why it is done Genetic testing is important for screening and sometimes medical treatment, as well as determining the risk of developing certain diseases. For a variety of reasons, various types of genetic testing are carried out:

Testing for diagnostics Genetic testing can tell you if you have the suspected disorder if you have symptoms that may be caused by genetic changes, also known as mutated genes. To confirm a diagnosis of Huntington's disease or cystic fibrosis, for instance, genetic testing may be utilized.

**Presymptomatic and prescient testing**. Getting genetic testing before you experience symptoms may reveal whether you are at risk of developing a genetic condition if you have a family history of that condition. For instance, this kind of test might be helpful for distinguishing your gamble of specific sorts of colorectal malignant growth.

**Transporter testing.** In the event that you have a family background of a hereditary problem — like sickle cell pallor or cystic fibrosis — or you're in an ethnic gathering that has a high gamble of a particular hereditary issue, you might decide to have hereditary testing prior to having kids. An expanded carrier screening test can determine if you and your partner are carriers for the same conditions by identifying genes linked to a wide range of genetic diseases and mutations.

**Pharmacogenetics.** This kind of genetic testing may assist in determining which medication and dosage will be most beneficial to you in the event that you suffer from a specific illness or condition.

**Pre-birth testing.** There are a few different kinds of genetic abnormalities that can be found during pregnancy through tests. Down condition and trisomy 18 condition are two hereditary problems that are frequently evaluated for as a feature of pre-birth hereditary testing. Traditionally, this was accomplished through invasive procedures like amniocentesis or by examining blood markers. Cell-free DNA testing is a new method that uses a blood test on the mother to examine the DNA of the baby.

**Screening for infants.** The most prevalent form of genetic testing is this one. In the, all of us states expect that babies be tried for specific hereditary and metabolic anomalies that cause explicit circumstances. This kind of genetic testing is important because, if the results show that a person has a condition like phenylketonuria (PKU), sickle cell disease, or congenital hypothyroidism, treatment can start right away.

**Testing prior to conception.** This test, also known as preimplantation genetic diagnosis, can be used to try to conceive via in vitro fertilization. The undeveloped organisms are evaluated for hereditary irregularities. In the hope of achieving pregnancy, unaffected embryos are implanted in the uterus. Risks

Generally, there are few physical risks associated with genetic tests. There is almost no risk with blood and cheek swab tests. Amniocentesis and chorionic villus sampling, however, carry a small risk of pregnancy loss (miscarriage).

Hereditary testing can have profound, social and monetary dangers also. Before having a genetic test, talk to your doctor, a medical geneticist, or a genetic counselor about all the benefits and risks involved.

**How to get ready:** Find out as much as you can about your family's medical history before you have genetic testing. To learn more about your risk, discuss your personal and family medical history with your doctor or genetic counselor. Clarify pressing issues and examine any worries about hereditary testing at that gathering. Also talk about your choices based on the results of the test.

If you're going to have genetic testing to see if you have a genetic disorder that runs in your family, you might want to talk about it with your family. You can get a sense of how your family might react to your test results and how it might affect them by having these conversations prior to testing.

Genetic testing is not covered by every health insurance policy. Therefore, before getting a genetic test, check with your insurance company to see if it will cover the costs.

The Genetic Information Nondiscrimination Act of 2008 (GINA) helps keep health insurers and employers from treating you unfairly because of your test results in the United States. Employment discrimination based on genetic risk is also against the law under GINA. Life insurance, long-term care insurance, and disability insurance are not covered by this act. Most states offer extra insurance.

What to expect? A sample of your blood, skin, amniotic fluid, or other tissue will be taken and sent to a lab for analysis, depending on the type of test.

**Blood Test.** An individual from your medical care group takes the example by embedding a needle into a vein in your arm. By pricking your baby's heel, a blood sample is taken for newborn screening tests.

**Swab of the Cheeks.** A swab from the inside of your cheek is taken for genetic testing for some tests.

**Amniocentesis.** A thin, hollow needle is inserted through your abdominal wall and into your uterus to collect a small amount of amniotic fluid for this prenatal genetic test.

**Sampling of Chorionic Villus.** For this pre-birth hereditary test, your PCP takes a tissue test from the placenta. The sample may be taken through your cervix with a catheter or through your abdominal wall and uterus with a fine needle, depending on your circumstance.

## Results

The timing of your genetic test results depends on the type of test and the health care facility you use. Converse with your PCP, clinical geneticist or hereditary guide before the test about when you can anticipate the outcomes and have a conversation about them.

## Positive Outcomes

Assuming the hereditary experimental outcome is positive, that implies the hereditary change that was being tried for was identified. Your next steps will be determined by the reason you underwent genetic testing in the first place.

If the intention is to:

A positive diagnosis of a specific disease or condition will assist you and your physician in selecting the appropriate treatment and management strategy.

If a test shows that you carry a gene that could cause a disease in your child, your doctor, medical geneticist, or genetic counselor can assist you in determining your child's likelihood of actually developing the condition. The experimental outcomes can likewise give data to consider as you and your accomplice go with family arranging choices.

Check to see if you might get a particular illness; a positive test does not necessarily mean you will get that illness. For instance, having a bosom disease quality (BRCA1 or BRCA2) implies you're at high gamble of creating bosom malignant growth sooner or later in your life, however it doesn't show with conviction that you'll get bosom disease. Nonetheless, for certain circumstances, like Huntington's sickness, having the changed quality demonstrates that the infection will ultimately create.

Discuss the implications of a positive result with your doctor. At times, you can make way of life changes that might decrease your gamble of fostering an illness, regardless of whether you have a quality that makes you more vulnerable to a problem. Additionally, the results may assist you in making decisions about treatment, career options, insurance coverage, and family planning.

You also have the option of participating in genetic disorder or condition-related research or registries. You might find that these choices help you keep up with the latest developments in treatment or prevention.

## Negative Results

A negative result indicates that the test did not find a mutated gene, which can be comforting but does not guarantee that you do not have the disorder. The precision of hereditary tests to recognize transformed qualities shifts, contingent upon the condition being tried for and whether the quality transformation was recently distinguished in a relative.

Even if you do not possess the mutated gene, this does not guarantee that you will never develop the disease. For instance, most people who get breast cancer don't have a gene for the disease (BRCA1 or BRCA2). Additionally, not all genetic defects may be detected by genetic testing.

Results that are not conclusive In some instances, a genetic test may not provide any useful information regarding the gene in question. Gene expression varies from person to person, but these variations typically have no effect on health. However, it can be challenging to tell the difference between a harmless gene variation and a gene that causes disease. Variants of uncertain significance are the names given to these alterations. In these instances, additional testing or periodic gene reviews over time may be required.

# Genetic Counseling

You should discuss any questions or concerns you may have with your doctor, medical geneticist, or genetic counselor regardless of the results of your genetic testing. This will assist you in comprehending the implications of the results for you and your family.

Changes in your DNA, also known as mutations or variants, are the focus of genetic testing. The medical care you or a member of your family receives can be altered by genetic testing, which is useful in numerous medical fields. For instance, genetic testing can provide information about your risk of developing cancer or a diagnosis for a genetic condition like Fragile X. Genetic tests come in many different varieties. A spit or blood sample is used for genetic testing, which typically yields results within a few weeks. If you are found to have a genetic change, your family members may also have the same change because we share DNA with them. Hereditary guiding when hereditary testing can assist with ensuring that you are the ideal individual in your family to get a hereditary test, you're getting the right hereditary test, and that you grasp your outcomes.

**Reasons to Get Genetic Testing:** To find out if you have a genetic condition that runs in your family before you have symptoms; to find out how likely it is that a current or future pregnancy will have a genetic condition; to diagnose a genetic condition if you or your child has symptoms; to understand and help you plan your cancer prevention or treatment. It could be for a number of reasons, including the fact that it is out of your reach or won't affect your medical care, that it is too expensive, or that the results could cause you anxiety or worry.

Different types of genetic tests Direct-to-consumer (DTC) genetic tests, which can provide some information about medical and non-medical traits, are distinct from clinical genetic tests. Your doctor will order clinical genetic tests for a specific medical reason. Healthy individuals who are interested in learning more about traits like ancestry, medication responses, or the risk of developing particular complex conditions typically purchase DTC tests. DTC test results can be utilized to arrive at conclusions about way of life decisions or furnish issues to examine with your PCP. However, you should not rely solely on DTC tests to make decisions about your treatment or medical care because they are unable to definitively determine whether or not you will contract a disease.

Genetic tests come in many different varieties. There is no one genetic test that is capable of identifying all genetic conditions. The way to deal with hereditary testing is individualized in view of your clinical and family ancestry and what condition you're being tried for.

**Testing a Single Gene.** One gene at a time is the focus of single gene tests. Single quality testing is done when your PCP accepts you or your kid have side effects of a particular condition or disorder. A few instances of this are Duchene solid dystrophy or sickle cell illness. Additionally, when a family has a known genetic mutation, single gene testing is utilized.

**Board Testing.** In a single test, a panel genetic test looks for changes in many genes. Hereditary testing boards are normally assembled in classes in light of various types of clinical worries. Low muscle tone, short stature, and epilepsy are all examples of genetic panel tests. Genes that are all linked to an increased risk of certain types of cancer, like breast or colorectal (colon) cancer, can also be grouped together in panel genetic tests.

Enormous scope hereditary or genomic testing. There are two various types of enormous scope hereditary tests.

Exome sequencing takes a gander at every one of the qualities in the DNA (entire exome) or simply the qualities that are connected with ailments (clinical exome).

The most extensive genetic test, genome sequencing examines all of a person's DNA rather than just their genes.

Doctors order exome and genome sequencing for patients with complicated medical histories. In addition, large-scale genomic testing is utilized in research to acquire additional information regarding the genetic causes of conditions. Secondary findings are results from large-scale genetic tests that have nothing to do with the reason the test was ordered in the first place. When looking for a genetic explanation for a child's developmental disabilities, secondary findings include genes linked to a risk of cancer or rare heart conditions.

Chromosome testing for changes other than gene changes. Chromosomes are the structures in which DNA is packaged. Instead of looking for changes in genes, some tests look for changes in chromosomes. Karyotype and chromosomal microarrays are two such tests.

## Expression of Genes

In various cell types, genes are turned on or expressed at various levels. Because knowing the difference between healthy and diseased cells can provide crucial information for disease treatment, gene expression tests compare these levels. These tests, for instance, can be utilized to direct breast cancer chemotherapy treatment.

**Types of Genetic Test Results Positive:** The test identified a known disease-causing genetic change.

Negative: there was no known genetic change found by the test. When the wrong test was ordered or there is no genetic cause for a person's symptoms, a negative result may occur. A "genuine pessimistic" is when there is a known hereditary change in the family and the individual tried didn't acquire it. A negative test result may not provide you with a definitive answer because there is no known genetic change in your family. This is due to the possibility that you were not tested for the genetic mutation that runs in your family.

Uncertain: A variant of unknown or uncertain significance indicates that there is insufficient information regarding the genetic change to determine whether it is pathogenic (causes disease) or benign (normal). An effective method for contemplating hereditary testing is as though you're posing the DNA an inquiry. We don't always find an answer because we didn't ask the right questions or because science doesn't yet know the answer.

**Next Steps:** Discuss with your doctor whether genetic testing is right for you if you have symptoms of a genetic condition, have a family history of a genetic condition, or are interested in learning more about your chance of having a genetic condition.

Diabetes raises the likelihood of developing chronic kidney disease. In order to assess your kidney health, your doctor may recommend one or more kidney tests. The sooner you know the soundness of your kidneys, the sooner you can do whatever it may take to safeguard them. Learn about these tests and what your results might mean—knowledge is power.

A condition known as chronic kidney disease (CKD) occurs when the kidneys become damaged over time and are unable to filter blood as effectively as they should. Diabetes is a major contributor to CKD, which typically does not present with symptoms until the kidneys are severely damaged.

The good news is that early detection and treatment of kidney disease may prevent CKD from getting worse and other health issues like heart disease. However, getting tested is the only way to determine how well your kidneys function.

If you have diabetes, you are aware of how crucial it is to avoid problems like CKD. Your kidney health will be examined by your doctor, typically through blood and urine tests.

Tests for Urine One of the earliest indications of kidney disease is proteinuria, or the presence of protein in the urine. A urine test will be ordered by your doctor to see if there is protein in your urine. There are two kinds of protein levels in your urine tests.

## Urine Dipstick Test

This test can be performed as a quick one to check for albumin, a protein produced by your liver, in your urine or as part of a comprehensive urinalysis. Although it does not offer a precise measurement of albumin, it does inform your physician that your levels are normal. A dipstick (a synthetically treated paper) is set in a pee test you give and in the event that levels are better than average, the dipstick changes tone. Assuming you have strange egg whites levels, your primary care physician might need to run further tests.

ratio of albumin to creatinine in the urine (UACR). This test measures the amount of albumin in your urine and compares it to the amount of creatinine, a waste product produced by the body's normal use and tear of muscles. A UACR test tells the specialist how much egg whites ignores into your pee a 24-hour time frame. Kidney disease may be apparent if the albumin level in your urine is above 30.

## It Is Critical To Know That:

To confirm the results, the test may be repeated once or twice.

In the event that you truly do have kidney sickness, how much egg whites in your pee assists your PCP with knowing which therapy is best for you.

A pee egg whites level that remains something similar or goes down implies that your treatment is working.

A doctor will also use a blood test to check your kidney function because your kidneys remove waste, toxins, and extra fluid from the blood. The results of your blood tests will indicate how efficiently and effectively your kidneys are eliminating waste. The following are a couple of blood tests that are utilized:

**Creatine in the blood.** The amount of creatinine in your blood is determined by a serum creatinine test. Your serum creatinine level will rise if your kidneys are not functioning as they should. Your gender, age, and the amount of muscle mass in your body will determine your normal levels.

Typically a creatinine level more than 1.2 for ladies and more than 1.4 for men might be an indication that the kidneys are not working like they ought to. Your doctor may want to conduct additional tests if the results of your serum creatinine test are higher than normal.

**Rate of glomerular filtration (GFR).** Your kidneys' ability to remove waste, toxins, and extra fluid from your blood is measured by your GFR. Your GFR is determined by taking into account your age, gender, and serum creatinine level. A normal GFR number for you will depend on your age and gender, just like it does with other kidney tests. In the event that your GFR is low, your kidneys are possible not functioning as they ought to. GFR decreases as kidney disease progresses. The aftereffects of your test can mean the accompanying:

In the event that you have a GFR number of at least 60 along with an ordinary pee egg whites test, you are in the typical reach. However, you should still talk to your doctor about when you should have another checkup.

If your GFR is less than 60, it could indicate kidney disease. You should talk to your doctor about the best treatment options for you.

If your GFR is less than 15, it could indicate that your kidneys are failing. You will most likely require dialysis or a kidney transplant if your results indicate kidney failure. You should be aware that your doctor may consider you for a kidney transplant as a precaution if your GFR level consistently falls below 20 over a 6- to 12-month period.

Blood urea nitrogen (BUN). The amount of urea nitrogen in your blood is measured by this test. Your body produces urea nitrogen as a byproduct of the breakdown of food protein. Urea nitrogen is eliminated from the body through the urine by healthy kidneys. This cycle assists keep your BUN with evening out inside a typical reach. Urea nitrogen levels typically range from 7 to 20 depending on age and any other health conditions you may have. Your kidneys may not be functioning as well as they should if your levels are higher than normal. Your BUN level rises with the progression of kidney disease.

Your doctor will use the results of your BUN test and other tests to determine the best course of treatment for you if your BUN level indicates kidney disease.

## Other Tests

Your doctor may also want to keep an eye on your blood pressure and suggest additional tests to look for kidney problems, like imaging or a biopsy.

## Pressure in the Body

Your doctor will want to keep an eye on your blood pressure because high blood pressure is one of the leading factors that lead to kidney disease and kidney failure. If you have CKD, controlling your cholesterol, blood sugar, and high blood pressure—all of which raise your risk of heart disease and stroke—is very important.

**Imaging.** These tests are utilized to get an image of the kidney to search for any issues or harm. Your doctor can see if there is a blockage or narrowing in the blood vessels or how well blood is flowing to your kidneys through imaging tests.

**Kidney Biopsy.** A kidney biopsy is a strategy where a little piece of kidney tissue is eliminated and inspected under a magnifying lens for indications of harm or infection. A thin needle is inserted through the skin to accomplish this.

Keep Your Kidneys Healthy By eating well, moving around, and keeping your blood pressure and cholesterol in the right range, you can lower your risk of CKD or prevent it from getting worse. Make a point to deal with your kidneys on the off chance that you are in danger for CKD. In the event that you have diabetes, get tried for kidney sickness once every year. Having your kidneys checked routinely allows you the best opportunity for finding and treating CKD early.

Tests and Diagnoses for Chronic Kidney Disease How Can I Tell If I Have It?

Most of the time, early kidney disease has no symptoms. The only way to find out how well your kidneys are working is through testing. Get checked for kidney infection assuming that you have

diabetes

hypertension

coronary illness

a family background of kidney disappointment

Assuming you have diabetes, get actually looked at each year. In the event that you have hypertension, coronary illness, or a family background of kidney disappointment, talk with your medical services supplier about how frequently you ought to get tried. The sooner you are diagnosed with kidney disease, the sooner you can receive treatment to aid in kidney protection.

How are kidney disease diagnoses and follow-ups determined by doctors?

A blood test called GFR, which measures how well your kidneys are filtering your blood, is used by doctors to look for kidney disease. The glomerular filtration rate is referred to as GFR.

a test for albumin in the urine. When the kidneys are damaged, they can release a protein called albumin into the urine.

In the event that you have kidney illness, your medical services supplier will utilize similar two tests to assist with checking your kidney sickness and ensure your therapy plan is working.